Anke Rüsbüldt

Horse Anatomy

Easy-to-understand and comprehensive

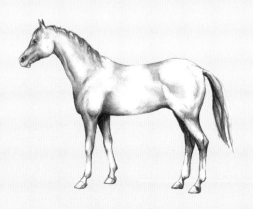

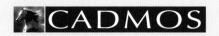

Contents

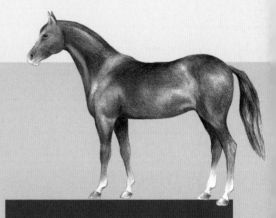

Imprint

Copyright © 2005 by
Cadmos Verlag GmbH, Brunsbek.
Translated by Ute Weyer
Layout and design: Ravenstein, Verden
Photography: Ende, Hoppe
Illustrations: Denmann
Printing: Rasch, Bramsche

ISBN 3-86127-951-7

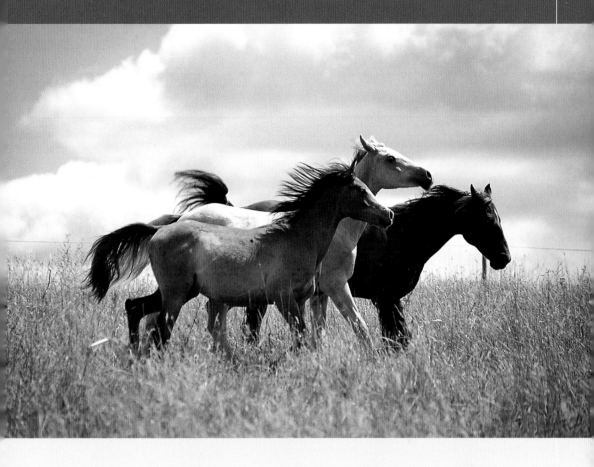

Why do you need anatomy?

Anatomy is the science that is concerned with the shape and structure of the body. In every situation in life, structure and function influence each other. The structure determines the function (a rectangular shape does not roll very well) and the function determines the shape (if we roll something long enough it becomes rounder). Anyone who wants to understand his or her horse should like to know how it functions. Even if someone only wants to ride, they still use the horse's functions. The structure of the horse, that is its anatomy, forms the basis for the function.

It is an advantage that not too many technical terms are needed to understand anatomy, but more a spatial awareness. Many structures can be felt and thus be learned. As horses are also mammals, many parts of their bodies are very similar to ours.

The aim of this book is to explain the basics – so that horse lovers see, understand and appreciate how wonderfully the equine body is put together, enabling it to fulfil its function.

We should remember that modern horses developed throughout the millenniums. Their ancestors were small omnivores. The specialised herbivorous flight animals of today developed much later. The skeleton still shows rudiments of once important structures that the horse needed for its long term survival. Adaptation through use by humans has, so to speak, only just begun. Many structures that are no longer needed are still present within the equine body.

3

Veterinary jargon

Veterinary surgeons all over the world talk about anatomy in Latin. Each structure has its own Latin name that vets have to learn at vet school. Riders, trainers and judges have their own technical terms too. In order to make mutual understanding easier, both parties should avoid these technical expressions whenever possible. Some terms however will be introduced here, as you will need to know them to discuss anatomy. You will also find some Latin words as they are now widely used by riders and in equine magazines.

Body sections:
The body of a horse can be roughly divided into forehand, middle and hindquarters. Everything from head to shoulders including front legs, belongs to the forehand; everything behind the flank to the hindquarters. The part in between – which is responsible for breathing, carrying and digestion – is the middle.

Directions:
We cannot avoid a bit of Latin here.
– Backward or towards the tail is called caudal.
– Forward or towards the head is called cranial.
– From the ears towards the nose is called rostral
– Upwards or towards the back is called dorsal. This applies to the legs as well.
– Downwards or towards the belly is called ventral.

This is different for the legs: for the front legs, palmar is used (towards the palm of the hand) and for the hind legs, plantar (towards the sole of the foot). A direction towards the middle is called medial and towards the side, lateral.

In addition to that, a structure close to the rump is proximal and away from the rump, distal. Using these expressions, an exact description of, for example, a bone, is now possible. If someone mentions the palmar side on a distal part of the cannon bone you will know what they are talking about.

Body parts:
These are quite simple and in some cases even called the same, for example: head, neck, shoulders, chest, abdomen, back, flank. Then on the front legs: upper arm, forearm, knee, and the hind legs: hip, upper thigh, heel.

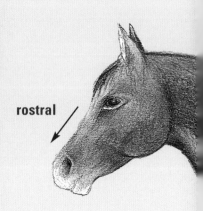

Forehan

rostral

dors

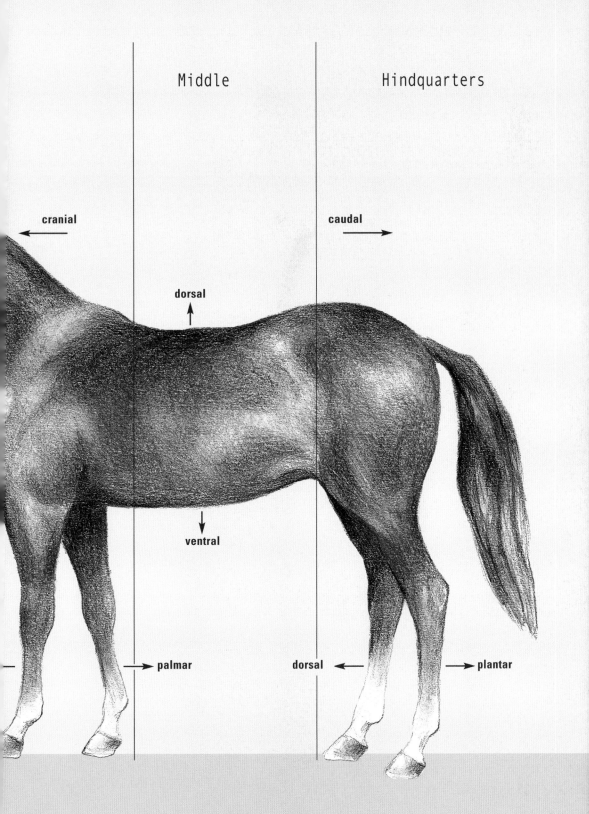

Middle

Hindquarters

cranial

caudal

dorsal

ventral

palmar

dorsal

plantar

What is where?

On the right you will find an overview of the anatomical structure of a horse.

If comparing the equine anatomy to that of a human, the equivalent joint to the human knee is the stifle, located at the top of the hind legs. The horse cannot flex his hock without also flexing the stifle and hip joints. In equine terms the forearm is above the knee (carpal joint) and the upper arm, above the elbow and all four points of the anatomy are in the forelegs.

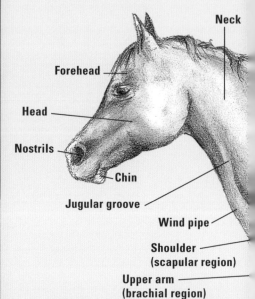

Neck

Forehead

Head

Nostrils

Chin

Jugular groove

Wind pipe

Shoulder (scapular region)

Upper arm (brachial region)

Breast

Knee

Cannon bone

Coronary band

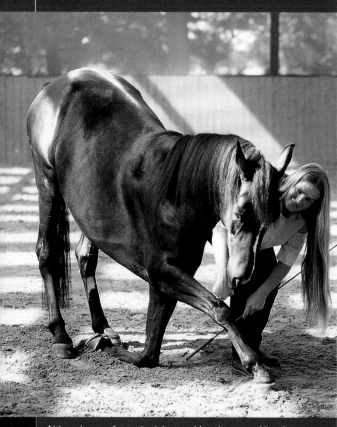

Although we refer to the joint touching the ground in a bow as the knee, the horse's joint that is the equivalent to the human knee is the stifle, located at the top of the hind legs where they join the trunk.

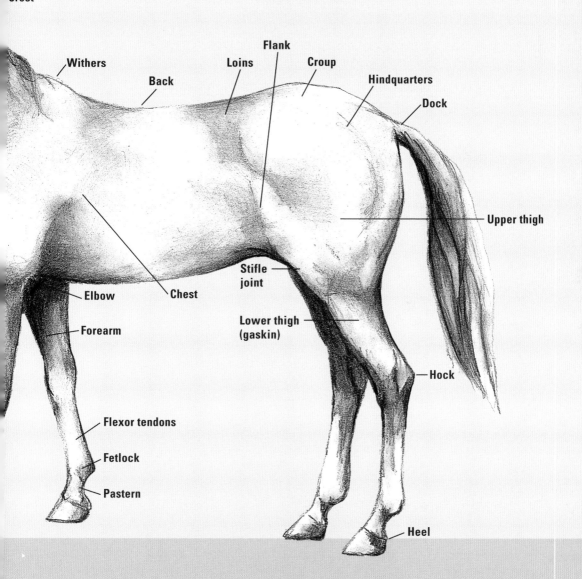

Crest

Withers

Back

Flank

Loins

Croup

Hindquarters

Dock

Upper thigh

Stifle joint

Elbow

Chest

Lower thigh (gaskin)

Forearm

Hock

Flexor tendons

Fetlock

Pastern

Heel

The skeleton

All mammals have a skeleton. They need it for stability and shape. It protects vital organs and enables movement.

The skeletons of mammals are all quite similar. For example, almost all mammals have seven neck vertebrae including humans, as well as horses and giraffes. These vertebrae, however, differ in size and shape.

The differences between the limbs of humans, that need to carry out very precise movements and manual skills, and those of horses, that require speed, are significant. The bones, however, are almost identical. Horses walk on the equivalent of the fingernail of our middle finger (or the hoof, in which the pedal bone is located). The splint bones, which are situated on either side of the cannon bones, and the chestnuts, on the insides of the legs above the hock and knee, are rudimentary structures from a time when the horse used to walk on several toes.

Another significant difference can be seen on the skull. In order to eat and chew plants, the horse requires very different teeth from us (see 'What does a horse need for eating?'). Also, it does not need as much brain in relation to its body weight. Being a flight animal, it requires large eyes with a wide-angle view (see 'The senses'). The equine skeleton developed to accommodate these requirements. The points of the skeleton that can be felt are marked here in yellow. You can feel these parts easily on a horse. However, do not forget that horses are easily frightened or can be ticklish and therefore be careful.

The bones are connected by joints. The type of joint determines the available movement, which can be a simple flexion as well as rotation or shifting.

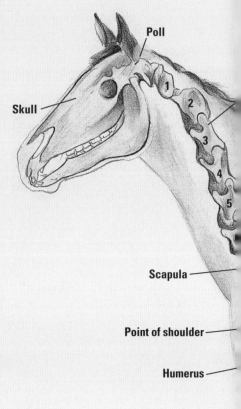

Poll

Skull

1
2
3
4
5

Scapula

Point of shoulder

Humerus

Radius

Cannon bone

Long pastern bone

Short pastern bone

Pedal bone

Neck (cervical) vertebrae (1–7)

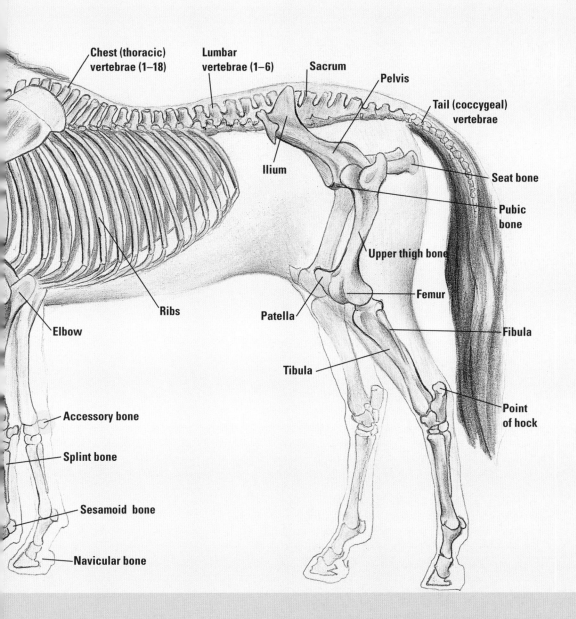

Chest (thoracic) vertebrae (1–18)

Lumbar vertebrae (1–6)

Sacrum

Pelvis

Tail (coccygeal) vertebrae

Ilium

Seat bone

Pubic bone

Upper thigh bone

Femur

Ribs

Patella

Fibula

Elbow

Tibula

Point of hock

Accessory bone

Splint bone

Sesamoid bone

Navicular bone

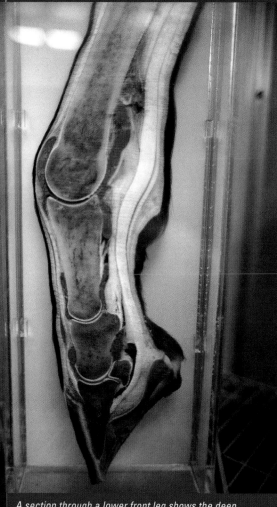

A section through a lower front leg shows the deep flexor tendon, which inserts at the pedal bone.

The Superficial Muscles

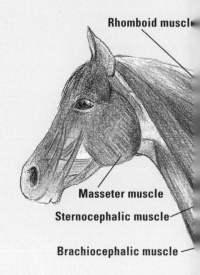

Rhomboid muscle

Masseter muscle

Sternocephalic muscle

Brachiocephalic muscle

Deltoid muscle —

Pectoral muscles —

Triceps muscle —

Extensor muscles —

The muscles

Skin muscles are situated immediately under the skin and they twitch involuntarily, for example, when an insect sits on the skin. Below them, separated by a thin layer of connective tissue, are the superficial muscles.

All muscles have points of insertion (see page 11). They contract when they work. Most muscles then shorten and bring the attachment sites closer together. This results in movement of connected bones. These functions determi-ne the muscles' names: stifle extensors, stifle flexors. Most muscles have an opponent (anta-gonist). Some muscles, for example the flexors of the lower limbs, move several joints at the same time. Others have various functions. A muscle that brings the front leg forward can also lower the neck when the horse is standing on that leg. Many muscles originate from a bone and end in a tendon that inserts at anot-her bone.

A horse can move his entire front leg using the muscles around the upper and lower thighs, there are no muscles below the knee, just ten-dons. Tendons form the ends of many strong

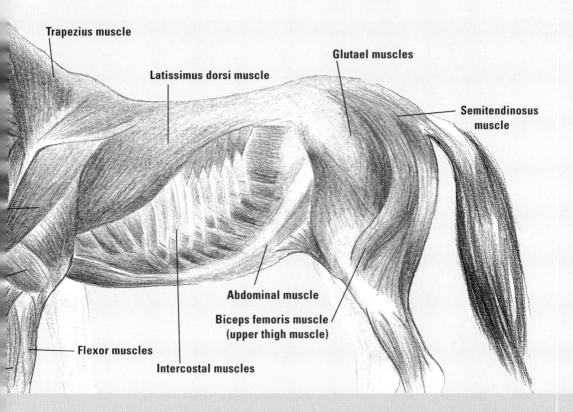

Splenius muscle

Trapezius muscle

Latissimus dorsi muscle

Glutael muscles

Semitendinosus muscle

Abdominal muscle

Biceps femoris muscle
(upper thigh muscle)

Flexor muscles

Intercostal muscles

flexor or extensor muscles and they are attached at certain bones. This is called insertion – an important word as diseases affecting these areas are called insertion desmopathy (desmo – ligament, pathy – illness). Parts of tendons that are subjected to a lot of pressure have an underlying bursa, this can be thought of as a small balloon filled with liquid.

Most muscles are paired, i.e. there is one on the left and one on the right side of the body. Often, their shape and symmetry shows whether one side works harder than the other. For example, when looking at a horse from behind, asymmetric rump muscles can sometimes be noted.

For muscles to work, they need to be stimulated by a nerve impulse. Depending on its function, a nerve can command all flexor muscles of a leg to contract. It is also possible that a nerve stimulates only one muscle. The regulation of movement is quite complicated and requires the precise interaction of many functions. The nervous system needs to obtain information about the actual movement required and will then send an impulse to the appropriate muscle or its opponent. Within a fraction of a second, feedback about the change in movement and about the position of, for example a limb, is sent back; the next impulse then follows. The exact structure and complex functions of the central and peripheral nervous systems are too complex to be discussed here.

The illustrations on pages 10–15 show the muscles of a horse. A selection of very large or very important muscles are described further below. Each muscle has at least one origin, one insertion site, one nerve and at least one function.

Shoulder and upper arm muscles

The triceps muscle (m. triceps brachii) is divided into three upper sections and originates from the posterior edge of the shoulder blade and two areas of the upper arm. It inserts at the elbow. The radialis nerve supplies its impulse. It extends the elbow and can also flex the shoulder joint.

The biceps muscle (m. biceps brachii) originates from the shoulder blade, inserts at the ulna and is supplied by the nervus musculocutaneous. This muscle flexes the elbow, extends the shoulder joint and can (via two merging tendons) stabilise the knee.

The deltoid muscle (m. deltoideus) originates from a tendinous area that is the equivalent of our collarbone, and from the shoulder blade. It inserts at the upper arm and is supplied by the nervus axillaris. It brings the front leg forward and can flex the shoulder joint.

Flexors and extensors of the front leg

The superficial flexor muscle (m. flexor digitalis superficialis) originates from the upper arm and inserts at the back of the pastern and the distal fetlock bone. It is supplied by the nervus ulnaris and flexes the knee and lower limb.

The deep flexor muscle (m. flexor digitalis profundus) has three origins: from the upper arm, the elbow and the middle of the forearm. It inserts at the back of the pedal bone and is supplied by the nervus ulnaris and nervus medianus. It flexes the toe.

The flexor tendons can be easily felt between the knee and fetlock when picking up the leg. Underneath them, close to the cannon bone, you also find the suspensory ligament. It is mainly tendinous and originates from the back of the cannon bone. It splits and inserts on each sesamoid bone.

The extensor muscle (m. extensor digitalis communis) originates from the upper arm and inserts at all three toe (phalanx) bones. The

The deep muscles

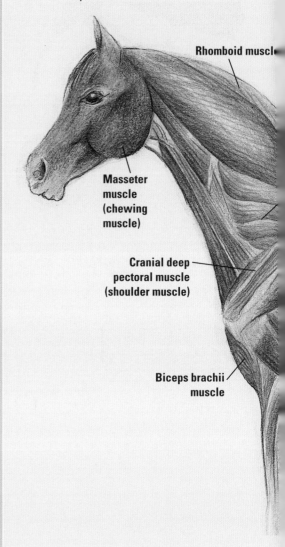

Rhomboid muscle

Masseter muscle (chewing muscle)

Cranial deep pectoral muscle (shoulder muscle)

Biceps brachii muscle

nervus radialis supplies this muscle which extends the toe. The extensor tendon can be felt on the front of the cannon bone.

The flexors and extensors of the hind leg are very similar.

Rump muscles

There are four rump muscles (m. glutaei) that originate from different parts of the hipbone and sacrum. They insert at the upper thigh and are supplied by the anterior and posterior ner-

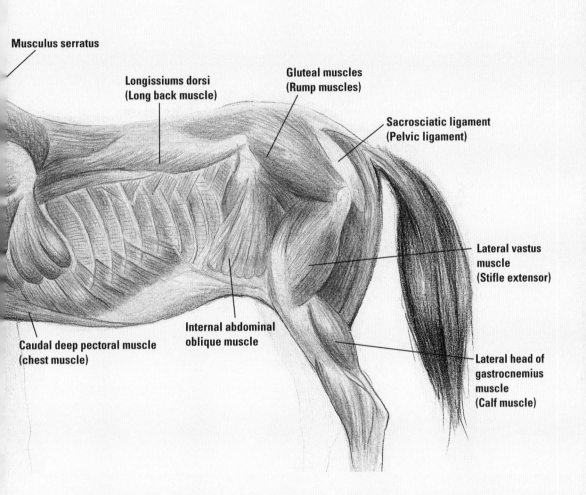

Musculus serratus

**Longissiums dorsi
(Long back muscle)**

**Gluteal muscles
(Rump muscles)**

**Sacrosciatic ligament
(Pelvic ligament)**

**Lateral vastus
muscle
(Stifle extensor)**

**Internal abdominal
oblique muscle**

**Caudal deep pectoral muscle
(chest muscle)**

**Lateral head of
gastrocnemius
muscle
(Calf muscle)**

vus glutaeus. They flex and extend the hip joint and can bring the hind leg forward and outward.

Long seatbone muscles
The two-headed upper thigh muscle (m. biceps femoris) originates from the lumbar vertebrae, the pelvic ligament and hipbone. It inserts together with the lateral and middle knee cap ligaments at the front of the lower thighbone. Its nerves are the posterior nervus glutaeus

and nervus tibialis. It extends the hip joint, stifle and hock.

The semitendinous muscle (m. semitendinosus) has similar origins and insertions as the biceps femoris, and on the weight-bearing leg it has a similar function. On the non weight-bearing leg it flexes the stifle and can move the leg inwards and backwards.

The muscles responsible for carrying and breathing are described in their respective chapters.

View from the front of the horse

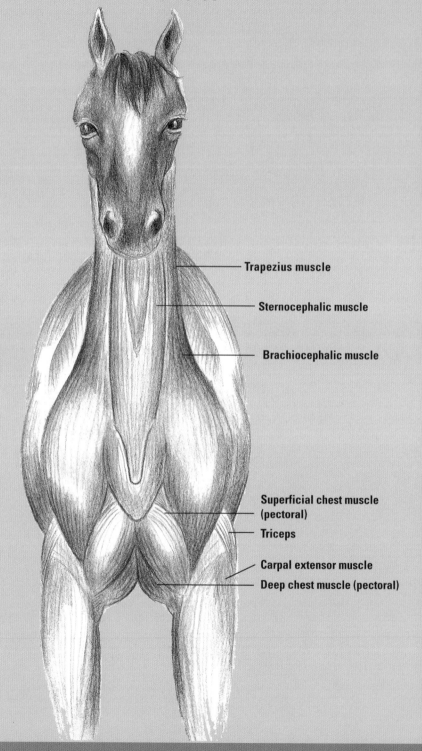

Trapezius muscle

Sternocephalic muscle

Brachiocephalic muscle

Superficial chest muscle (pectoral)

Triceps

Carpal extensor muscle

Deep chest muscle (pectoral)

View from above the horse

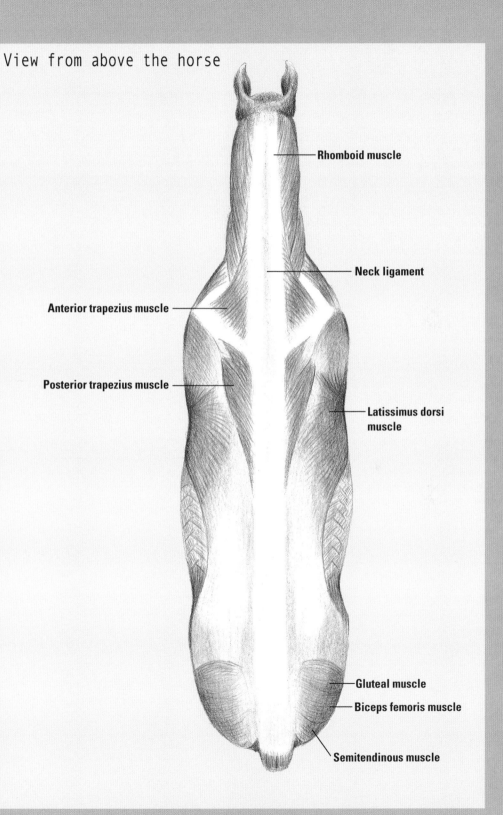

Rhomboid muscle

Neck ligament

Anterior trapezius muscle

Posterior trapezius muscle

Latissimus dorsi muscle

Gluteal muscle

Biceps femoris muscle

Semitendinous muscle

How does a horse carry its rider?

The spine acts like a bridge with the legs being pillars. In order for a horse to carry a rider, this bridge has to bend upwards. It is a wide misconception that only the back muscles are responsible for this. The action of the abdominal muscles are also very important!

Abdominal muscles follow four different directions and all of them meet in a tendinous structure along the midline. When pressing this tendon with your finger, a healthy horse will automatically arch its back. The abdominal muscles are also used to support the breathing. Their action is easily visible on an exhausted horse or one suffering from chronic lung disease. Thickening of the abdominal muscles forms a groove while the tendinous area does not change.

The neck ligament is also very important for carrying a rider. This ligament originates from the back of the skull and attaches with a segment at each of the neck vertebrae. It then carries on along the back across all the vertebrae. When a horse lowers its head, it arches its back. Many back or neck problems stem from a weak or tense neck ligament caused by incorrect riding.

The detailed picture of the toe shows the pedal bone, which supports the horse's weight, and its attachment to the sensitive layer in the foot. This attachment is very effective, as it has to carry the whole mass of the horse. Now take a look at your own fingers: the horse walks on the fingernail of the middle finger. The attachment of the bone in the foot is so good because the sensitive layers in the hoof that cover the pedal bone have many branches. These form a close network of fine laminae that becomes visible at the white line on the sole. If these laminae were flattened out they would cover an area as large as a football pitch.

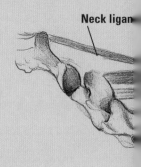

Neck ligament

Hoof wall

White line

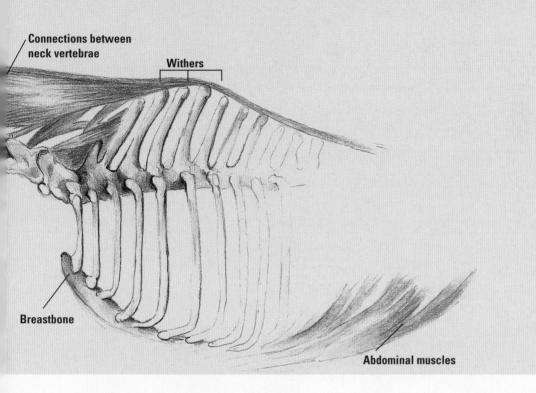

Connections between
neck vertebrae

Withers

Breastbone

Abdominal muscles

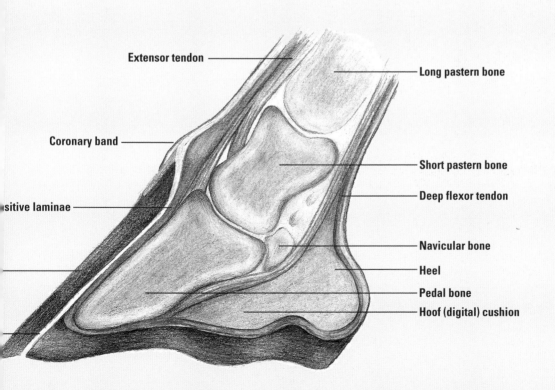

Extensor tendon

Long pastern bone

Coronary band

Short pastern bone

Deep flexor tendon

sitive laminae

Navicular bone

Heel

Pedal bone

Hoof (digital) cushion

What does a horse need for breathing?

First of all, a horse needs to have breathing muscles. The most important one is the diaphragm. This muscle has a tendinous part in the middle and separates the chest cavity from the abdomen. The diaphragm is shaped like a vault and advances into the chest cavity. During inspiration, it flattens without changing the position of the most anterior tip. This creates more room in the chest and the lungs can extend along the chest walls. During expiration, the elastic lungs allow the air to escape again while the diaphragm returns to the shape of a vault. Between the lungs and the chest walls lies the so-called pleura. This consists of two very thin tissue layers with a small amount of fluid in between. The effect is similar to two layers of cling film with a drop of liquid between them. You can move them against each other but not separate them as long as no air can get in between them. This system helps attach the lungs to the inside of the chest cavity.

There are also muscles between the ribs that pull the ribs forwards and upwards during inspiration and backwards and inwards during expiration. Parts of the abdominal muscles also function as supportive breathing muscles.

When a horse breathes in, air flows through the nostrils into the nasal passages. These are lined with a mucus membrane and the air is warmed up and cleaned. The air then continues to the larynx and trachea. The larynx makes sure that food travels into the oesophagus and air into the trachea. You can feel the cartilage of larynx and trachea along the lower part of the neck. (Be careful, horses do not like this very much.)

The trachea divides into two bronchi that then branch out into smaller bronchioli and finally end as many small bubbles (alveoli). The latter are surrounded by a fine network of blood vessels. After inspiration the exchange of gasses takes place here. Used carbon dioxide is removed from the blood into the alveoli and oxygen is moved from the alveoli into the blood stream.

Photo of the lungs of a horse

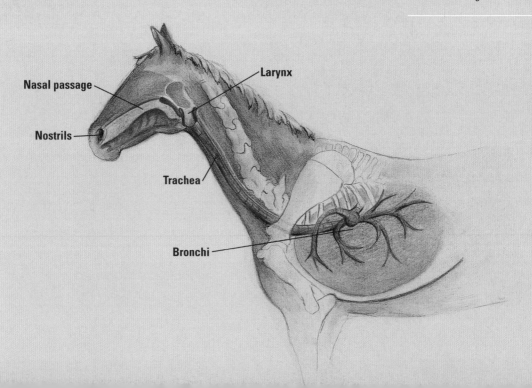

Larynx

Nasal passage

Nostrils

Trachea

Bronchi

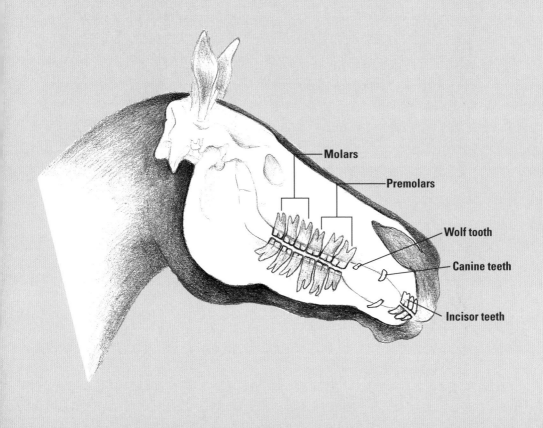

Molars

Premolars

Wolf tooth

Canine teeth

Incisor teeth

What does a horse need for eating?

First of all, a horse needs teeth for eating. Like us, horses develop milk teeth to start with that later fall out and are replaced by permanent teeth. Equine permanent teeth, however, "grow" throughout almost all of their life. A new born foal usually only has two incisor teeth. By the age of twelve months it will have 24 teeth, and then the first permanent molars that have no deciduous predecessors will appear. At two and a half years, the exchange of teeth begins and will be complete at about four and a half years. The permanent teeth will have developed their final shape at the age of about six years. Permanent teeth have certain patterns on the chewing surfaces (tables) depending on

the age of the horse. The shape of the tables changes with age as well, from oval to triangular to elliptical. The angle of the incisors in the jaw becomes flatter with time. Twice in a horse's life, the position of upper and lower jaw changes so that the third incisors develop a groove on the outside.

All these changes help the expert to age a horse. There are some differences between breeds, however, and other factors (vices like crib biting or excessive wear as well as necessary tooth treatments) can lead to false estimations.

Apart from the thirty-six permanent teeth, some horses have additional teeth. Between the incisors and premolars of the lower as well as upper jaw, canine teeth (also called "tushes") can appear. Some horses also have a small tooth in front of the first upper, and rarely the lower, premolar called a wolf tooth. These sometimes interfere with the bit and, if so, should be removed.

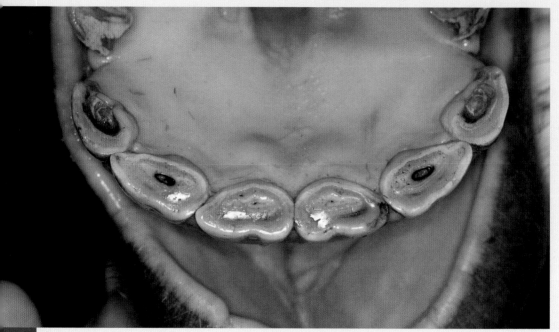

The cups on the inner incisor tables of this horse have disappeared.

Easy to spot: hooks along the outside of the premolars and molars and a wolf tooth.

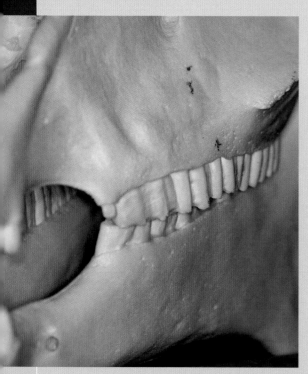

Horses tear out grass with their incisors. They do not bite it off, they grab the grass and move their heads to tear it off. The grass is then pushed between the molars where it is broken down and chewed. The upper and lower jaws need to enable movement of the teeth backwards and forwards as well as sideways. Irregular teeth or uneven wear leads to the development of hooks that make efficient chewing impossible. Horse's teeth should be checked regularly every six months or yearly, and then be treated if necessary. Malfunctioning teeth can lead to colic, tension, riding and back problems.

The roots of the upper premolars and molars reach up into the sinuses. In the case of a tooth root infection, a badly smelling nasal discharge usually occurs.

The teeth developed throughout evolution to be able to graze poor, hardy grassland. As the food available to horses nowadays has changed, it is important to check these "wrongly used" teeth regularly and have them treated as required.

Incisor teeth of a five year old horse:

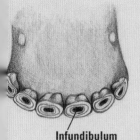

Infundibulum

Incisor teeth of a horse more than 20 years old

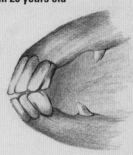

Jaw in a cross section:

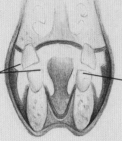

Possibility of appearance of unwanted hooks

Chewing surface

Longitudinal section through an incisor tooth of a five year old horse

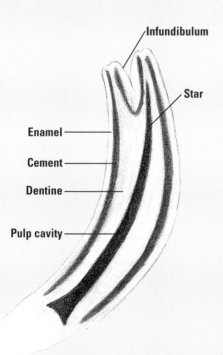

Infundibulum

Star

Enamel

Cement

Dentine

Pulp cavity

Cross section of the chewing table shows the age related changes created by wear

5 years

Star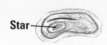
8 years

11 years

13 years

20 years

21

What does a horse need for digestion?

After chewing the food thoroughly and mixing it with saliva, it is then swallowed. The food passes the larynx and reaches the oesophagus. This muscular tube transports it to the entrance of the stomach. It is sometimes possible to see the food move through the oesophagus when looking at the left side of the horse's neck. Insufficiently chewed food, dry sugar beet, or bigger hard particles (small apples, beetroot, carrots) can lead to an obstruction of the oesophagus. This can be life threatening! There are three areas within the oesophagus that are particularly narrow and therefore prone to obstructions: at the entrance to the chest, above the heart and at the entrance to the stomach.

If chewed and swallowed properly, the food reaches the stomach. The entrance into the stomach is such that food can pass in only one direction – it is true that horses cannot vomit. There is another danger: a stomach can be overloaded! An equine stomach can only hold up to twelve litres. Five litres of quickly eaten food can be too much.

From the stomach, the food is moved into the small intestines. They are divided into three parts, are over twenty-six metres long and are the central area of digestion. The first part immediately following the stomach is called the duodenum. Juices produced by the pancreas and bile from the liver are added to the food here. The liver is situated on the right side within the chest area. Horses, like humans, produce bile which is very important for digestion, but they have no gall bladder to hold the bile – a popular trick question.

After passing through the small intestines, the food reaches the caecum. This large organ lies on the right side in the flank area and can hold about thirty litres. Its entrance is located at the top of the right flank, the "hunger groove" – an area that sinks inwards when a horse is very thin. The caecum is not visible but can be heard at work if you hold your ear against the horse's belly. About twice every three minutes you can hear that typical noise when food is pushed from the small intestines into the caecum. The food is now fermented and further digested with the help of bacteria. It then moves on to the large intestines where bacteria help extract more nutrients that are absor-

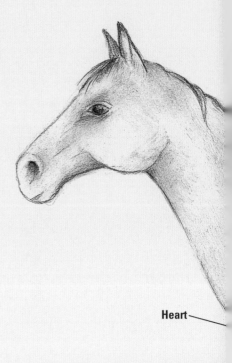

Heart

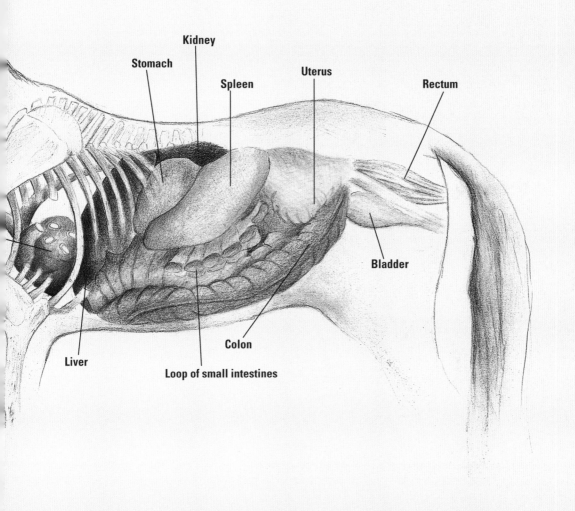

Kidney

Stomach

Spleen

Uterus

Rectum

Bladder

Liver

Colon

Loop of small intestines

bed through the intestinal walls. The colon is also many metres long and is folded in two layers either side of the abdomen. Its last part predominantly reabsorbs fluid from the digested food. The food moves through the rectum and is passed through the anus as well shaped droppings.

The horse's kidneys are situated outside of the peritoneum, roughly behind the last ribs, underneath the spine. They filter noxious substances and metabolic waste products from the blood and produce urine that flows through the kidneys and ureters into the bladder. From here, the urethra leads to the outside.

The circulatory system

Blood consists of about two thirds liquid with dissolved substances and one third cells. These are the white and red blood cells and platelets that are important for blood clotting.

Blood flows through the whole body and transports oxygen and nutrients to the tissues. On its return, it takes carbon dioxide and waste products with it.

The heart is a pump that constantly moves the blood. It has four chambers and is located in the lower chest cavity. Oxygenated blood passes through the left atrium into the left main chamber. It is then pushed through the aorta into the body. It reaches the neck and head via the carotid arteries. The aorta curves round towards the body and supplies all organs and muscles, via arteries, with blood. In the smallest arteries, called capillaries, oxygen exchange takes place. The blood is then transported back through veins. It reaches the heart via the superior and inferior vena cava. The carbon dioxide-rich blood travels through the right atrium into the right main chamber and via the pulmonary artery into the lungs. A fine network of capillaries in the lungs enables the gaseous exchange. The pulmonary vein transports the oxygenated blood back to the heart.

The interaction between ventricles and atriums works throughout the horse's entire life and without a break – that is the unique accomplishment of the heart muscle! It is the closing of the valves situated between the chambers that allows the pressure to build up and can be heard with a stethoscope.

When the blood is pumped across the body, it gets momentum from the heart. This can be felt as a pulse in various places along the legs. After passing the capillary network in the hoof this momentum is lost. The movement of the hoof creates new energy that helps push the blood back to the heart (and now uphill). The weightbearing hoof expands and the frog thrusts the blood upwards. Only regular and natural exercise can keep this mechanism going.

Illustration of the circulatory system

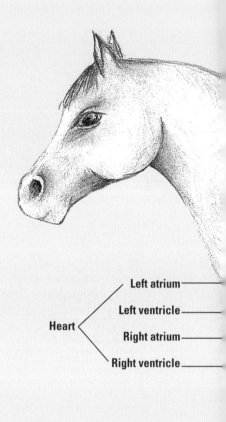

Heart
- Left atrium
- Left ventricle
- Right atrium
- Right ventricle

Pulmonary vein

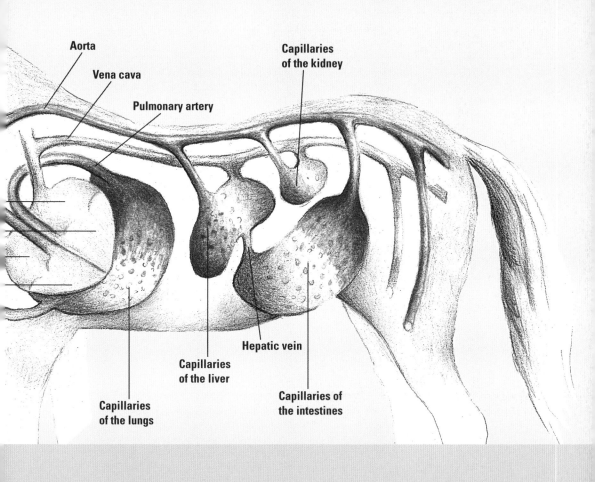

Aorta

Vena cava

Pulmonary artery

Capillaries
of the kidney

Hepatic vein

Capillaries
of the liver

Capillaries of
the intestines

Capillaries
of the lungs

The lymphatic system

The lymphatic system is protective as well as a waste removal system. It recovers tissue fluid and in the lymph nodes, which act as a kind of filter station, it recycles this fluid.

Lymph fluid is a light-coloured fluid consisting mainly of water. Salts, proteins and fat are dissolved in it as well as some blood cells.

The lymph vessels originate from all areas of the body as very fine branches and mostly run parallel to the veins. They collect excess and used fluid from the tissues. The main function of the lymphatic system is to support the body's immune system.

The lymph vessels lead to lymph nodes in which many white blood cells eliminate waste products.

If, for example, an infection on a limb develops, the circulation in this area starts to increase. More fluid is carried to the infected part that contains increased amounts of inflammatory products, cells and debris. The lymph vessels transport this fluid to the nearest lymph node where the waste products are filtered out and eliminated. The purified fluid then reaches the main lymph vessel in the abdomen and is pushed back into the blood vessels. The flow through lymph vessels is usually slow and is supported by the movement of the horse.

Prolonged rest can lead to congestion within the lymphatic system. The horse's legs swell up. As long as no other infectious problems are present that challenge the immune system, lymph drainage can be carried out. This specific type of massage can activate the lymph flow again.

Some lymph nodes can be felt. The mandibular lymph nodes lie between both sides of the lower jaw underneath the head. They are roughly walnut sized, fairly smooth and can be moved against the surrounding tissue. The lymph nodes near the parotid glands can be felt as well: food contains many harmful substances that are filtered out here before they can hurt the body.

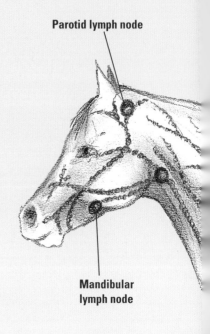

Parotid lymph node

Mandibular lymph node

In case of a massive infection, a lymph node may not be able to cope. It will then swell up and accumulate masses of pus inside until its walls cannot withstand the pressure any more. These lymph nodes feel large and warm at first, but can no longer be moved against the surrounding tissue and will finally burst open. This can happen, for example, on the lower jaw in connection with tooth problems, and not cause any significant illness. However, in the case of strangles, it can be very dramatic and involve large amounts of pus.

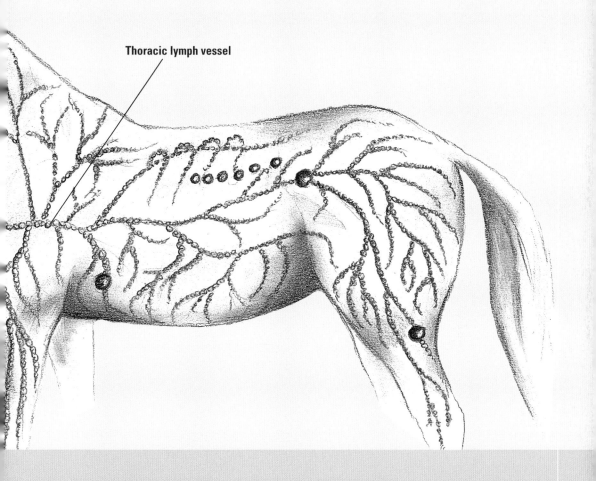

Thoracic lymph vessel

The reproductive system

The female horse, called a mare, is sexually mature at about eighteen months of age. Before putting a mare into foal, it is healthier to wait until she is fully grown and not before the age of three. The mare comes into season every three weeks and she is then fertile for a few days. Her ovaries produce follicles that contain an egg cell. The egg travels along the Fallopian tube towards the uterus. If the mare is covered at the correct time, the egg cell will be fertilised by sperm during this journey. The fertilised egg is then implanted into the uterus and undergoes cell divisions and grows. From day fourteen, the embryo can be detected by ultra sound. After eleven months and one week, the neonatal foal has grown sufficiently and is born through the widened cervix and vagina. These processes are triggered by certain hormones that can also be detected in the blood.

Where did the sperm come from? Sperm cells mature inside the stallions testicles. During mating, they are ejected through the erect penis together with fluids from the sexual glands. The sperm cells are deposited inside the mare's vagina. At many studs, it is common nowadays to collect sperm first in a glass tube, examine and dilute it and then inject it into the mare's uterus using insemination catheters.

During pregnancy, the mare's body undergoes changes. She deposits more fluid in her tissue and at the end of term the udder develops. Most brood mares tend to become fat, which is unhealthy and should be avoided.

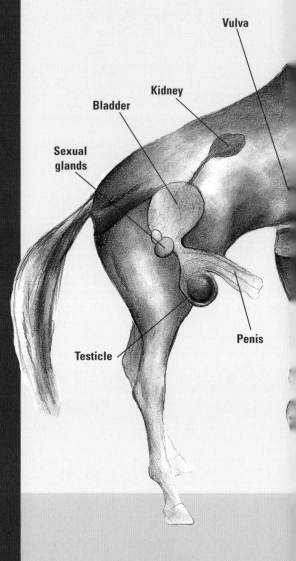

Vulva

Kidney

Bladder

Sexual glands

Penis

Testicle

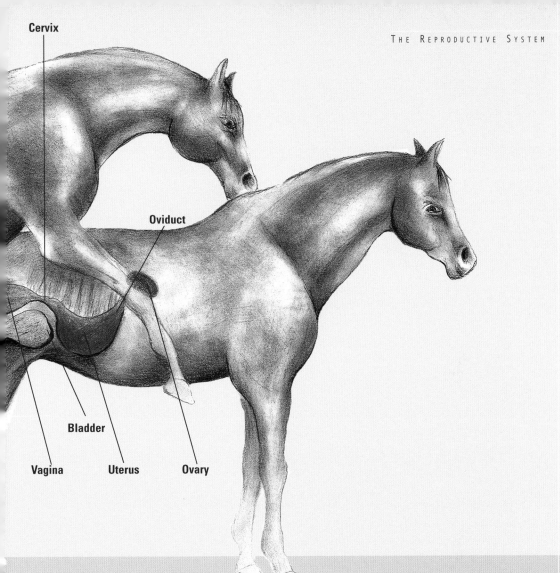

Cervix

Oviduct

Bladder

Vagina   Uterus   Ovary

Overview of the female sexual organs

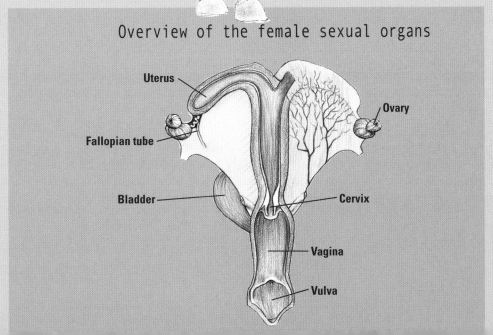

Uterus

Ovary

Fallopian tube

Bladder

Cervix

Vagina

Vulva

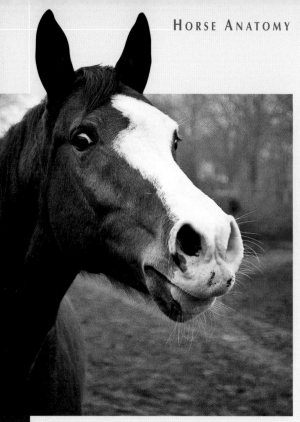

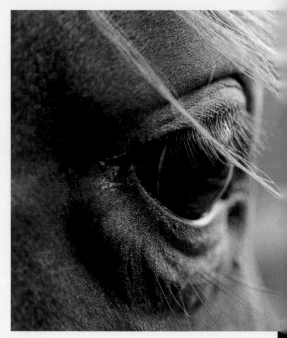

Using all senses to decide: flee or relax?

A calm eye contemplating the world

The senses

The horse is a flight animal and compared to us is the master of perception. It can detect the smallest movements from miles away. Its excellent view is facilitated by the location of the eyes with their long and pretty pupils far to the sides of the head. It can thus see everything around it without having to move its head apart from an area immediately ahead of and exactly behind it. The flexible neck further allows a perfect all-round view. Horses, however, are less capable of focussing on close objects and their spatial vision is inferior to ours.

Horses have small grape-like dark structures (corpora nigra) along the edges of the pupils. These nigra are normal parts of the retina and their most likely purpose is as a protection from very bright light. Horses see colours differently to us. They can distinguish yellow and blue better than red and green. Coloured show jumping fences of the same size

and width are therefore being judged differently by a horse.

Another, equally important sensual organ is the skin. A horse reacts very sensitively to insects. The lips with their tactile hairs and vast amounts of nerve endings can detect even the smallest food particles extremely well. Contrary to a cow for example, a horse would never eat a nail. The skin also serves as a thermo regulator. On cold days, the circulation of the skin is reduced and the hairs are erected in order to reduce heat loss. If the body needs to loose heat, the blood flow through the skin is increased and sweat is produced which leads to cooling through evaporation.

Now to the ears. Some horses resent having their ears touched. These large ears can be turned in all directions. Hearing is very sensitive and selective. The sounds travel through the outer ear towards the eardrum. In the middle and inner ear the sound is converted into nerve impulses that are recognised by the brain as certain noises. The inner ear is also the centre for balance. The ears play a part in the horse's body language. They are a valuable communication tool and indicate the horse's moods.

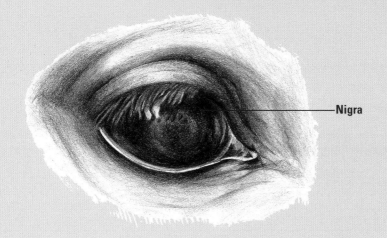

Nigra

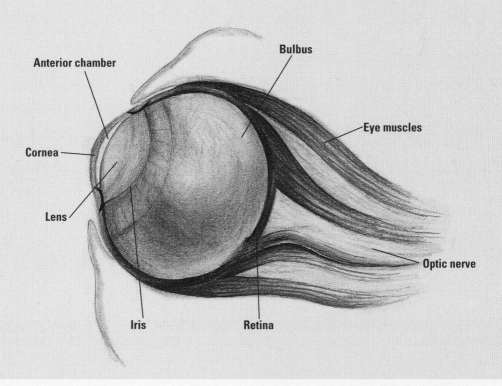

Anterior chamber

Bulbus

Eye muscles

Cornea

Lens

Optic nerve

Iris

Retina

There is little literature describing the horse's sense of taste. They probably have, like humans, taste buds on their tongue. Some horses can move their tongue well and can, for example, separate the stone of a plum and spit it out.

The horse's sense of smell is superior compared to that of humans. When a horse wants to intensify a certain smell it starts "flehmen", a lifting of its upper lip. A word of caution: some horses also show flehmen when they have abdominal pain.

Many equine books state, not for nothing, that the use of perfume should be avoided when dealing with horses. They regard strong artificial smells as aggressive and uncomfortable and their own perception is also compromised.

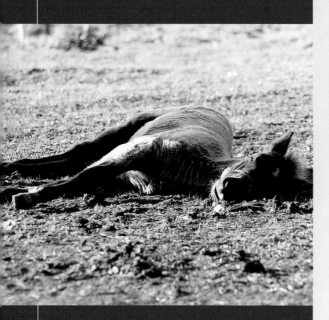

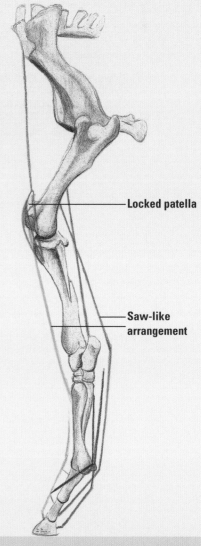

Locked patella

Saw-like arrangement

How does a horse sleep?

Horses can sleep in a relaxed and quiet manner, just like humans, while lying flat on the ground. Their sleeping patterns, however, are different from ours and they need less sleep than we do. Horses also dream when sleeping deeply. In order to be able to lie down, horses require a suitable surface and the feeling of security. Horses unable to sleep properly over a long period of time become ill and fractious. As an undisturbed sleep was not always possible for horses in the wild, nature was inventive: horses can also sleep while standing. Although this is more of a deep dozing rather than proper sleep, it nevertheless works and refreshes them.

This standing sleep is possible due to a locking mechanism in the legs. The joints are stabilised without having to rely on muscle power, due to the tendons and ligaments forming a kind of fixed frame around them. This works particularly well in the hind legs that require more stabilisation when standing due to their increased angles. When standing, the horse's patella is connected to the lower part of the femur by a loop of ligaments. It has to be pushed out of this fixation before the horse is able to walk. As long as the patella is fixated the whole leg is locked. As the special arrangement of muscles and ligaments between stifle and hock (like a double saw) allows only simultaneous movements of both joints, the locked stifle automatically locks the hocks as well. Therefore, horses can, when they sleep standing up, rest one hindleg while the body weight is distributed on three legs, without having to use muscle strength or having to concentrate on this.